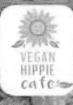

VEGAN HIPPIE SOL

Delicious Recipes for the Plant-Based Soul!

DOMINIQUE WILLIAMSON

Table Of Contents

VEGAN HIPPIE SOL:

DELICIOUS RECIPES FOR THE PLANT-BASED SOUL!

Chef and plant enthusiast, **Dominique Williamson** grew up in the deep south eating classic soul food such as biscuits and gravy, creamed corn, sweet mouth-watering cornbread, and tons of other classics. After going plant based Chef thought she would have to give all of her favorite dishes up until she found a way to veganize everything. Chef has spent countless hours, days, and nights experimenting in the kitchen and coming up with different ways to incorporate her southern roots with her plant-based diet. The outcome? A handful of recipes have now been designed and put on paper for all of the vegan hippies out there. Chef's first cookbook **VEGAN HIPPIE SOL** features smokin' sausage biscuits and gravy, BBQ pulled "pork' ' sandwich, philly cheez steaks, coconut creamed corn, sweet agave banana cornbread, and more. These recipes come from deep within and from generations back and most importantly a healthier alternative to childhood favorites. Grab your apron and let's get ready to cook! Enjoy!

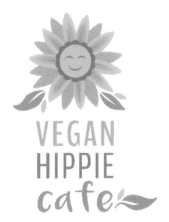

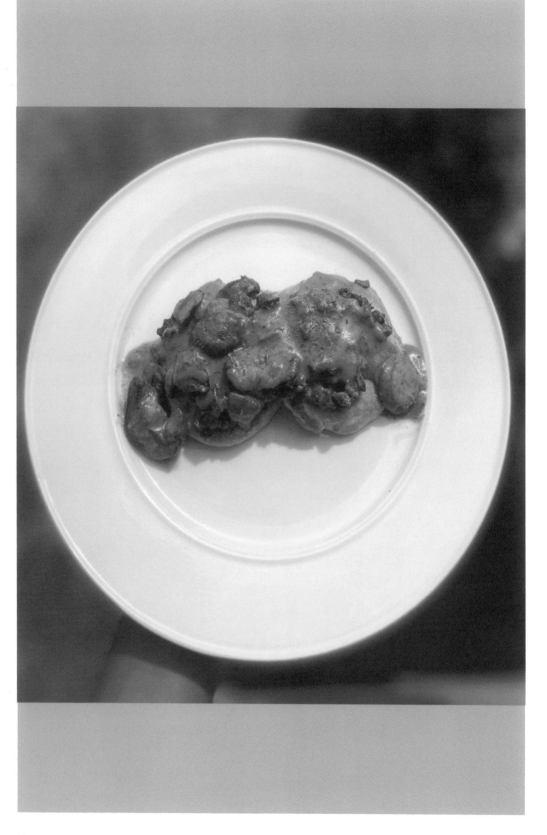

FLUFFY BUTTERMILK BISCUITS N GRAVY

PREP IN
15-25 minutes

READY IN
45 minutes

SERVES
6-8 people

TIPS

→ Place dough on parchment paper and then put it in the oven for better results.

→ Combine agave, melter butter, and cinnamon for agave butter.

→ If you do not have a rolling pin then use a wine bottle.

→ Don't over think. Cooking should be fun.

→ Curdled- separate or cause to separate into curds or lumps.

INGREDIENTS

→ 1 stick of earth balance butter

→ 2 ½ c. all-purpose flour

→ 1/2 tsp baking soda

→ 2 tsp baking powder

→ 1 tsp salt

→ 1 tbsp sugar

→ 1 c. non-dairy milk

→ 2 tbsp apple cider vinegar

PREPARATION

1. Combine flour and butter in a bowl. Use a potato masher to cut the butter into the flour until you reach a crumbly consistency. Once that consistency is reached add the remainder of your dry ingredients. Mix with your hands thoroughly. Place in the freezer.

2. Mix non-dairy milk and apple cider vinegar together and stir together. Set aside for five minutes or until curdled. (This will make your vegan butter milk).

3. Remove dry ingredients from the freezer and create a hole in the middle of the dough to add buttermilk. SLOWLY add buttermilk and mix everything together until you have a wet, but cohesive dough. (Add more flour if it gets too wet).

4. Place dough on a FLOURED surface and mold the dough until cohesive. When cohesive, roll the dough until it's 1-1.5 inch thick. Fold it into itself 4-5 times. After the fifth time roll it out again to about 1-1.5 inch thick.

5. Preheat the oven to 400 degrees. Take a floured cookie cutter and cut the dough to form biscuits. Place on a baking pan with parchment paper (if you don't have parchment paper just spray the pan with butter or oil).

6. Brush the top of biscuits with vegan butter and place in the oven for 20 minutes or until golden brown.

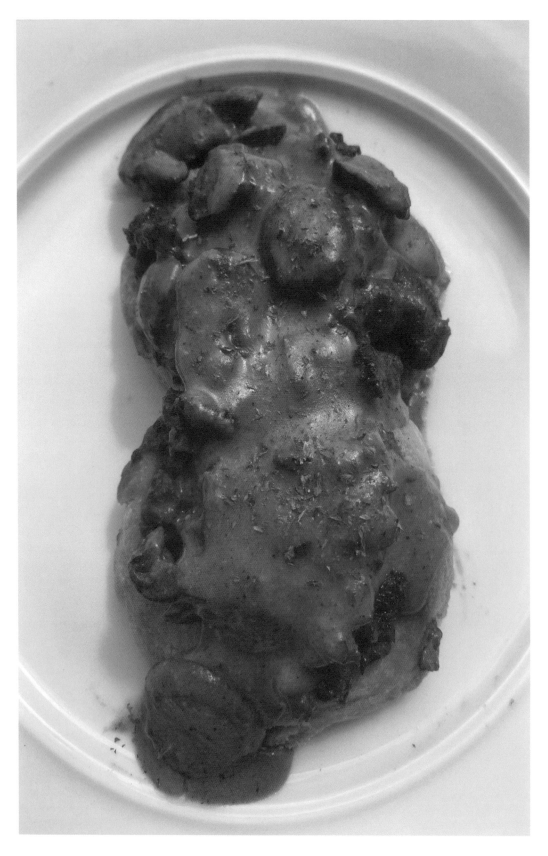

SMOKED SAUSAGE GRAVY

PREP IN
15 minutes

READY IN
25 minutes

SERVES
4 people

TIPS

- Don't over think. Cooking should be fun.
- Adjust seasonings to your liking.
- Mushrooms are a great substitute for a meat alternative.
- Don't over think. Cooking should be fun.

INGREDIENTS

- Half a pack of Beyond Beef ground beef
- 2 c. Portobello Mushrooms (sliced)
- 1 tbsp Earth Balance
- 1 c. non dairy milk
- 2 tbsp all-purpose flour
- 1 tbsp pepper
- 1 tbsp onion powder
- 1 tbsp garlic powder
- 1 tsp chili powder
- 1 tsp smoked paprika
- ⅛ tsp cayenne (optional)
- 1 tbsp brown sugar
- 1 tsp liquid smoke (optional)
- Salt to taste
- Chili flakes (optional)

PREPARATION

1. Heat up a sautéing or frying pan on medium-low heat. Add a drizzle of olive oil and a scoop of butter and spread to cover the pan. Add half of your beyond meat and use a spatula to break it up. until it looks similar to ground beef. Add a pinch of sea salt. Let it cook for 5-6 minutes.

2. Now, add the portobello mushrooms to the pan and turn heat to medium. Add all seasonings and mix together. Let cook for 5-6 mins.

3. Add flour and mix together. Coat everything in the pan. Let it cook for 60 seconds or until it resembles a roux.

4. Add COLD milk & stir. Adjust heat to medium/low. Over time the gravy will start to thicken up. Add another pinch or two of salt and pepper and liquid smoke.

5. Serve over biscuits and enjoy!

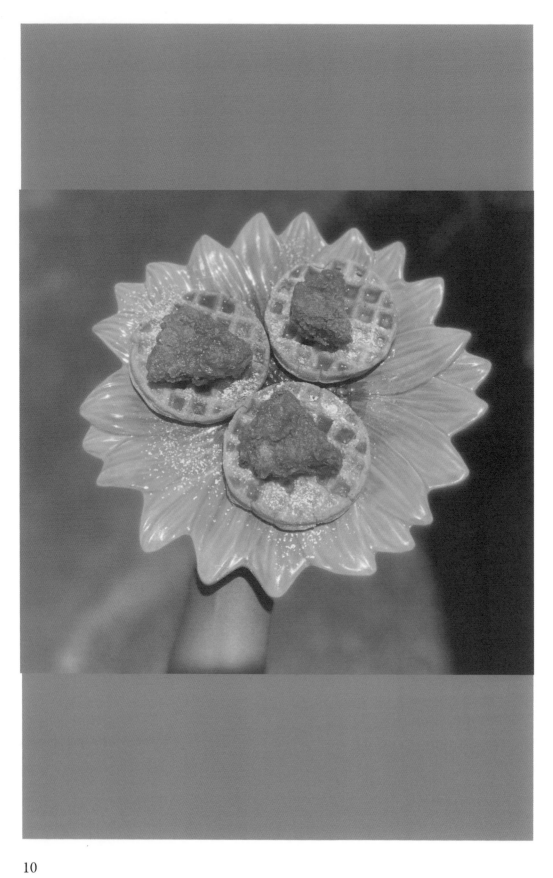

CHIKIN & WAFFLES

PREP IN

10 minutes

READY IN

15 minutes

SERVES

6 people

TIPS

➥ Best served with maple syrup.

➥ Adjust seasonings to your liking.

INGREDIENTS

➥ Refer to *Southern Fried Chikin recipe*

➥ 1 ¾ c. spelt flour

➥ 1 tsp baking powder

➥ ½ tsp baking soda

➥ 6 tbsp aquafaba

➥ 2 tsp vanilla

➥ 1 tsp cinnamon

➥ ¼ tsp nutmeg

➥ ¼ - ½ c. coconut sugar

➥ 1 ¾ c. Almond milk

➥ 1 tbsp vegetable oil

➥ 4 tbsp Earth balance

FOR SERVING

➥ Maple syrup

➥ Earth balance butter

PREPARATION

1. Refer to the Southern *Fried Chikin recipe.*

2. For the waffles, whisk together all of the dry ingredients in a large circular bowl.

3. Stir in wet ingredients until all ingredients are combined. The batter should resemble waffle mix/pancake mix.

4. Preheat waffle iron and brush with butter to prevent batter from sticking.

5. Ladle about ½ - ¾ cup of batter onto the waffle iron and cook until golden brown.

6. Repeat with the remaining batter.

7. Top with *fried chikin*.

8. Serve with maple syrup and seasonal fruit.

9. Enjoy!

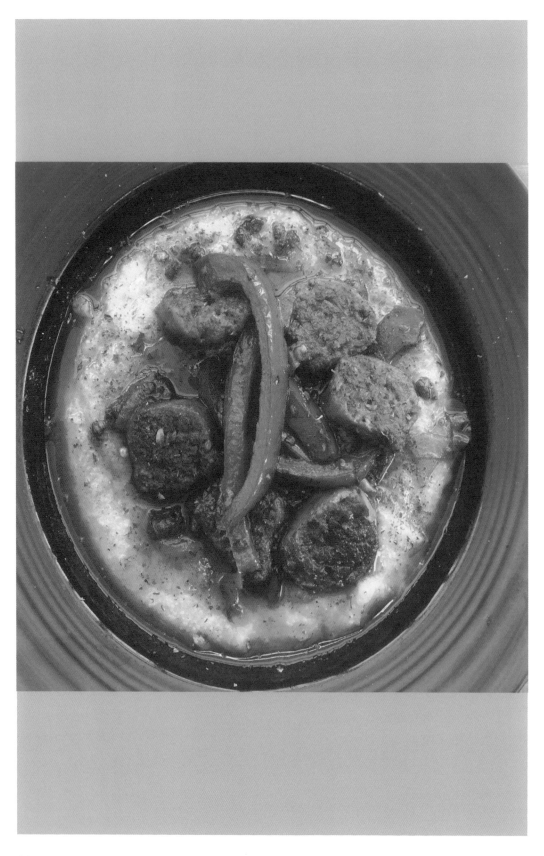

SOUTHERN LOADED CHEDDAR GRITS

PREP IN
10 minutes

READY IN
15-20 minutes

SERVES
3-4 people

TIPS

- You can use yellow or white grits.
- Do NOT use cornmeal that is used for baking things such as cornbread. Use GRITS!
- Adjust seasonings to your liking.
- Add more broth if you want a juicer sauce to put over grits.
- ALL Beyond Meat are 100% vegan.

INGREDIENTS

- 1 c. grits, coarse grind
- 4 c. vegetable broth
- 1 package Beyond Sausage
- 2 red peppers
- 2 green peppers
- 1 sweet onion, diced
- 1 package portobello mushrooms
- 2 tbsp nutritional yeast
- 1 tbsp garlic powder
- 1 tsp cajun seasoning
- 1 tsp old bay seasoning
- ½ tsp cayenne
- 2 tbsp vegan butter
- 1 tbsp olive oil.
- Healthy pinch of salt and pepper
- ¼ cup daiya cheddar cheese
- 2 garlic cloves, minced (optional)

PREPARATION

1. In a large non-stick pot bring 4 cups of vegetable broth to a boil. Add a pinch of salt and stir in grits.

2. Lower heat and simmer and cover. Cook for 20 minutes or until grits are tender. Season with nutritional yeast, salt, pepper, daiya cheese.

3. While the grits are cooking start prepping all vegetables and beyond sausage.

4. In a large saute pan on medium heat, add 1 tbsp of olive oil along with minced garlic. Let garlic cook for 20 seconds.

5. Add all vegetables in along with all of your leftover seasonings. Cook for 5 minutes and then add in sausage. Add in ⅛ cups vegetable broth and butter. Cook for another five minutes. Do not let all of the liquid evaporate. Keep the juices!

6. Once the vegetables are done serve over grits and enjoy! Season with more salt and pepper if needed.

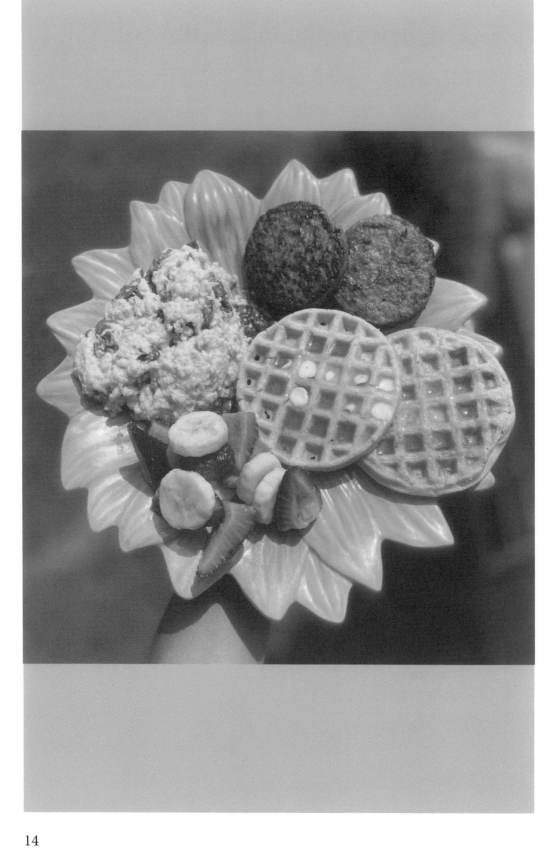

BEST VEGAN EGG SANDWICH

PREP IN
05 minutes

READY IN
20 minutes

SERVES
3 people

TIPS

→ Use Non-stick pan for best results.

→ Add spinach if you'd like.

→ Add nutritional yeast for a cheesy flavor.

→ It's important that you use a NON-STICK PAN!

→ Just Egg is made from mung beans which are packed with healthy nutrients and contains high antioxidant levels, which also reduces chronic diseases.

INGREDIENTS

→ 1 bottle of Just Egg

→ Vegan bread of your choice

→ 1 c. of white mushrooms

→ 1 sweet onion (chopped)

→ 2 tsp garlic powder

→ 1/4 tsp pepper

→ 1 tbsp of Earth Balance

FOR SERVING

→ Vegan Mayo

→ Salt for taste

→ Pepper flakes (optional)

→ 1 avocado, sliced

PREPARATION

1. Prep onions and mushrooms. Oil pan and cook until translucent.

2. Once translucent add half a bottle of JUST Egg along with seasonings. Quickly scramble.

3. Set vegan eggs to the side once finished or leave in a pan on LOW. Butter one side of your bread and toast on griddle for 2-3 mins. While the bread is toasting, slice avocado.

4. Remove bread from the griddle and on the BUTTERED side add your vegan mayo and avocado. Top with egg. Top with the other slice of bread.

5. Enjoy!

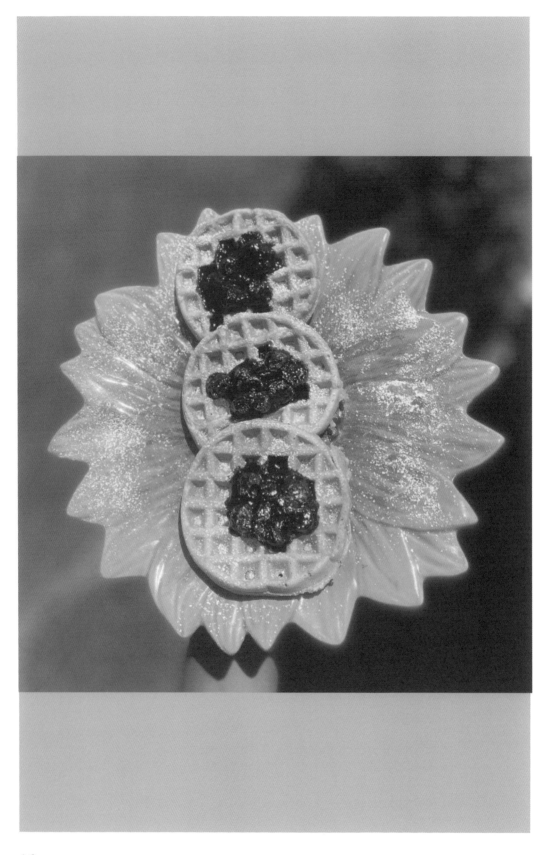

"BUTTERMILK" BLUEBERRY WAFFLES

PREP IN
05 minutes

READY IN
10 minutes

SERVES
6 people

TIPS

- Best served with maple syrup.
- Can substitute Apple Cider vinegar for lemon juice.
- Curdled: separate or cause to separate into curds or lumps.
- Blueberries are often called superfoods and help aid heart health!

INGREDIENTS

- 1 ¾ c. all-purpose flour
- 1 tsp baking powder
- ½ tsp baking soda
- 6 tbsp aquafaba
- 2 tsp vanilla
- ¼ - ½ c. coconut sugar
- 1 ¾ c. almond milk
- 1 tbsp lemon juice
- 1 tbsp vegetable oil
- 4 tbsp earth balance
- ½ c. blueberries

FOR SERVING

- Maple syrup
- Bananas, sliced
- Strawberries, sliced
- Blueberries

PREPARATION

1. Prep all ingredients.
2. Combine lemon juice with non-dairy milk. Set aside until curdled.
3. Whisk together all of the dry ingredients in a large circular bowl.
4. Stir in wet ingredients until all ingredients are combined. The batter should resemble waffle mix/pancake mix.
5. Stir in milk and blueberries.
6. Preheat waffle iron and brush with butter to prevent batter from sticking. It is important that the waffle iron remains on a medium setting to avoid burning blueberries.
7. Ladle about ½ - ¾ cup of waffle batter onto the waffle iron and cook until golden brown.
8. Repeat with the remaining batter.
9. Top with seasonal fruit and syrup.
10. Enjoy!

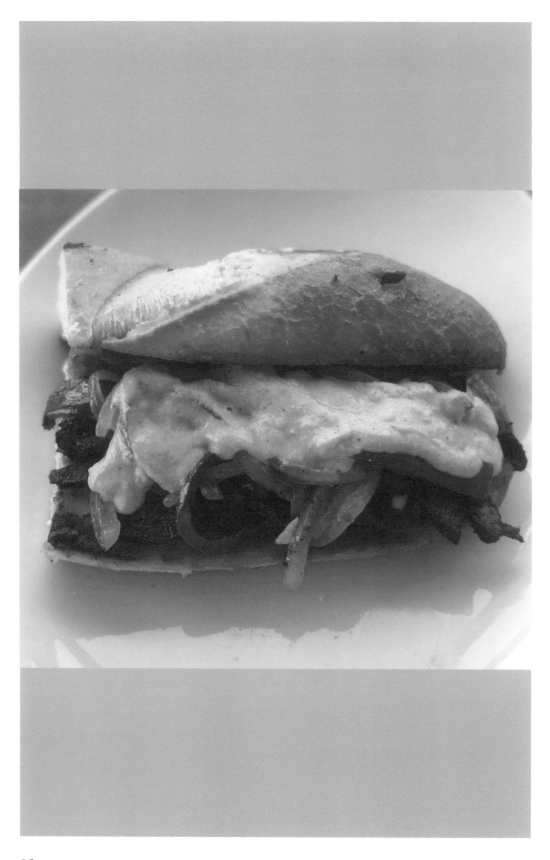

PHILLY CHEEZ STEAKS

PREP IN
20 minutes

READY IN
45 minutes

SERVES
4 people

TIPS

- Flash fry: fry (food) briefly and at a very high temperature.
- Oyster mushrooms can be used as a substitute for chanterelle mushrooms.
- Hoagie Rolls are recommended.
- Recommended seasonings: Vegan Steak seasoning, salt, pepper, garlic power, nutritional yeast.
- Most edible mushrooms contain Vitamin B which helps strengthen the immune system.
- Cashew cheese can help lower blood pressure and is an excellent choice of protein.

INGREDIENTS

- 1 yellow onion
- 1 green pepper, sliced
- 1 red pepper, sliced
- 1 c. cashews
- 3 c. of sliced portobello mushrooms
- 1 c. shiitake mushrooms
- 1 pack of chanterelle mushrooms
- 4 cloves of garlic, minced
- ½ - 1 c. vegetable stock
- ¼ c. daiya cheese
- 3 tbsp steak seasoning, vegan
- 1 tbsp garlic powder
- 1 tsp onion powder
- Salt and pepper to taste
- 1 tbsp liquid smoke
- Bread of your choice
- 1 tsp olive oil
- 1 tbsp earth balance

PREPARATION

1. Prep all of your vegetables. Preheat the oven to 400 degrees.
2. Oil cast iron skillet with olive oil.
3. In a medium cast iron skillet, place mushrooms in a pan and cook on medium/high 2 minutes on each side. The goal is to flash fry your mushrooms.
4. Season with onion powder, garlic powder, salt, pepper, steak seasoning (optional).
5. Finish off in the oven for 8-10 mins.
6. Heat skillet to medium heat and add earth balance, olive oil, and garlic.
7. Add in red pepper,green peppers, and onion. Add salt, pepper, garlic powder to taste.
8. After the veggies become translucent, add vegetable broth and turn heat to medium/high.
9. Let vegetable broth be reduced in half. Then turn off the burner.
10. Toast bread and then prepare your philly.
11. Add mushrooms, cheese sauce, onions and peppers.
12. Enjoy!

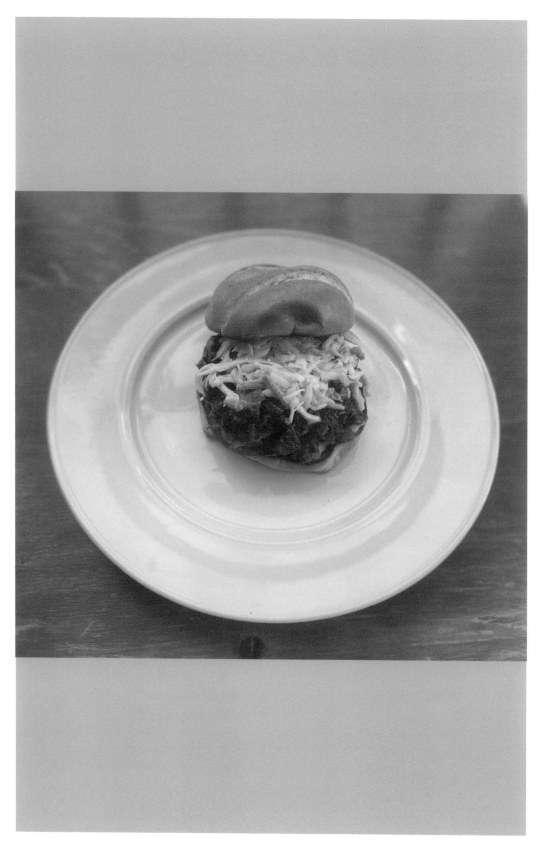

SMOKIN' PULLED PORK SAMMICH

PREP IN
25 minutes

READY IN
30 minutes

SERVES
3-4 people

TIPS

→ Adjust seasonings to your liking.
→ Grilled pineapple is optional, but delicious. Just take pineapple rings and sear for 2 minutes on each side.
→ Jackfruit can be subbed for mushrooms.
→ Cast iron skillet is recommended.
→ Oyster mushrooms are a great source for protein and are low in saturated fat!

INGREDIENTS

→ 3 medium sized king oyster mushrooms
→ 2 tbsp liquid smoke
→ 1 tsp smoked paprika
→ 1 tbsp chili powder
→ 2 tbsp garlic powder
→ 1 ½ tsp cayenne pepper
→ 1 tbsp onion powder
→ 1 tsp cumin
→ 1 tsp chili flakes (optional)
→ 3 garlic cloves finely minced
→ ½ c. bbq sauce (vegan)
→ 1 tbsp veggie broth
→ 1 tsp brown sugar (for sauce)

FOR SERVING

→ 4 whole wheat vegan buns
→ Grilled Pineapple (optional)
→ Vegan Mayonnaise
→ Purple Cabbage (finely chopped)

PREPARATION

1. Prep oyster mushrooms by taking a fork and shredding them to get thin sized strings. Similar to pulled pork.
2. In a mixing bowl add all dry seasonings, olive oil, and liquid smoke, and oyster mushrooms. Mix together and make sure mushrooms are well seasoned.
3. Place mushrooms in a cast iron skillet and place the oven on a broil setting (high).
4. Broil on high for 7 minutes.
5. In a saucepan combine BBQ sauce, minced garlic, brown sugar, and veggie broth. Whisk together on low heat. Add more BBQ sauce as needed.
6. Pull oyster mushrooms out of the oven and brush with BBQ sauce until evenly coated. Place back in the oven for another two minutes.
7. Broil until 90% of moisture is cooked out. If the mushrooms still look super wet then place back in and broil until 90% moisture is cooked out.
8. Toast buns and prepare to serve.
9. Place oyster mushrooms on the bun and top with grilled pineapple, purple cabbage, mayo and more vegan BBQ sauce.
10. Enjoy!

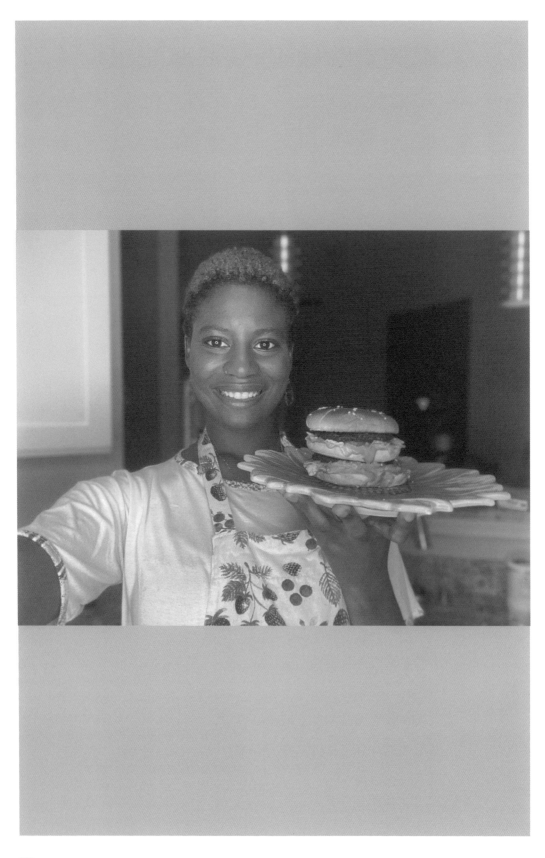

VEGAN BIG SMAC

PREP IN
5 minutes

READY IN
15 minutes

SERVES
1 person

TIPS

- Adjust seasonings to your liking.
- You can use both beyond patties if you want a meatier burger.
- If the Big Mac Sauce still tastes like mayo, add more ketchup and vinegar.
- If Big Mac Sauce is too thick add more plant milk or vinegar.
- If the Big Mac Sauce is too sour add more agave and plant-milk.

INGREDIENTS

- 1 Beyond meat patty
- 2 slices of vegan cheddar cheese
- Vegan hamburger buns
- 2 tbsp red onions, diced
- ⅛ cup iceberg lettuce
- Pickle chips for topping

- 1 tsp onion powder
- 1 tsp garlic powder
- ¼ tsp seasoning salt
- ¼ tsp paprika
- ½ tsp liquid smoke
- ¼ tsp cumin

BIG MAC SAUCE

- 2 tbsp vegan Mayo
- 1 tsp mustard
- 1 tsp sweet relish
- 1-2 tsp vinegar or apple cider vinegar
- 1-2 tbsp ketchup
- ½ tsp Agave
- 1 tsp plant milk
- Pinch of salt

PREPARATION

1. In a medium bowl combine beyond meat patty, dry seasonings, and liquid smoke. Set aside for 10 minutes.

2. Split the patties into two even balls and place them into an oiled pan on medium heat.

After cooking for 60 seconds gently flatten the patties. Cook on each side for 5-7 minutes or until crispy, but juicy.

3. Top each patty with vegan cheese and add 1 tbsp on water and cover. Turn the burner on low and the steam from the water will allow the cheese to melt.

4. In a small bowl combine all ingredients listed under **Big Mac Sauce.**

5. Put together the sandwich. To assemble the burgers, spread a little **Big Mac Sauce** over the bottom base. Top with some red onion, shredded lettuce, beef patty and some pickle slices. Top with the middle bun, and spread with more Big Mac sauce, onion, lettuce, pickles, beyond beef patty and then finish it off with more sauce. Top with top burger bun and serve. Garnish with sesame seeds.

6. Enjoy!

COCONUT CREAMED CORN

PREP IN
2 minutes

READY IN
8-10 minutes

SERVES
4-6 person

TIPS

- If you don't have arrowroot powder substitute with cornstarch.
- Use coconut milk for cooking, NOT for drinking.
- Coconut milk aids in weight loss and can strengthen the immune system.

INGREDIENTS

- 1 tbsp Earth Balance
- 3 c. sweet corn
- 1 tbsp ginger
- 1 tsp coconut sugar
- 1 ½ c. coconut milk
- 1 tsp arrowroot powder
- Salt for taste

PREPARATION

1. In a medium sized saucepan over medium heat combine vegan butter, ginger, salt and cook for 1 minute.

2. Add corn and sugar. Cook for 5 mins and stir frequently.

3. Reduce heat to low and add coconut milk.

4. Mix arrowroot powder and some coconut milk to get a liquid consistency. Add back into the pot. Let it simmer for 10 minutes. Check and stir frequently.

5. Once it has thickened up it is ready to serve. Enjoy!

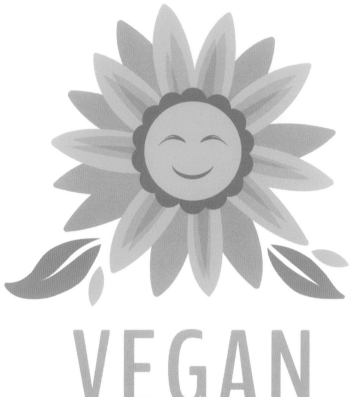

VEGAN
HIPPIE
sol

RED BEANS & RICE

PREP IN
15-25 minutes

READY IN
1 hour 30 mins

SERVES
4-6 person

TIPS

➥ Use a large non-stick pot.

➥ Food processor works best.

➥ Add field roast sausage for "meaty consistency".

INGREDIENTS

➥ 1 pound red kidney beans soaked or canned

➥ 1 medium yellow onion, diced

➥ 1 green bell pepper, diced

➥ 2 stalks of celery, diced

➥ 5 cloves of garlic, minced

➥ 32 ounce veggie broth

➥ Spoonful of Earth Balance

➥ 1-2 tbsp hot sauce

➥ 1 tbsp garlic powder

➥ 1 tsp thyme

➥ 1 tsp of pepper

➥ ⅛ tsp cayenne

➥ 1 ½ tsp paprika

➥ 3 bay leaves

➥ Salt to taste

➥ 1 tsp of liquid smoke (optional)

➥ 1 tbsp of crushed chili flakes (optional)

➥ 2 c. white or brown rice

PREPARATION

1. Place your earth balance, celery, onion, and green pepper in a large pot on medium until translucent. Once translucent, add minced garlic. Stir all ingredients together to ensure everything cooks evenly.

2. Add hot sauce, thyme, paprika, salt, pepper, garlic powder, and stir evenly to coat the vegetables. Let it cook on medium for 2-3 minutes.

3. Now add soaked kidney beans, vegetable broth, bay leaves, chili flakes to the pot and bring the temperature down to low. Place a lid on and let it reduce for 1 hour. Check often and stir every 15 minutes.

4. Once the beans have reduced, take ¼ cup of beans and pulse them in a food processor. Add back to the pot when finished. This step is very important because it allows for the beans to be creamy and have the right texture. **DO NOT SKIP THIS STEP.**

5. Add liquid smoke and simmer for an additional 10 mins.

6. Serve over rice and Enjoy!

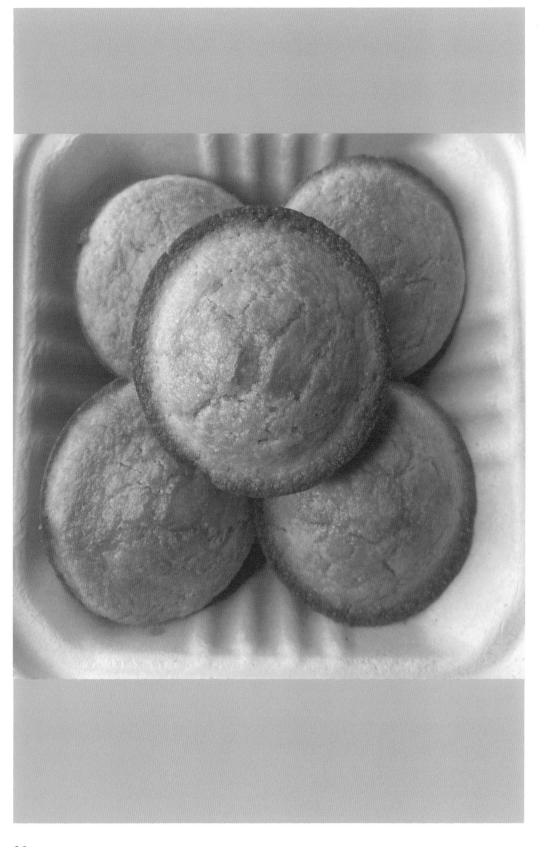

SWEET AGAVE CORNBREAD MUFFINS

PREP IN
10 minutes

READY IN
20 mins

SERVES
8 person

TIPS

- Use non-stick pan
- Combine dairy-free butter, agave, sugar, and cinnamon for sweet butter.
- Bananas are optional.
- Bananas aid in digestion and can also provide you with energy.

INGREDIENTS

- 1 c. flour
- 1 c. cornmeal yellow maíz
- 1/4 c. sugar
- 4 tsp baking powder
- 1 c. almond milk
- 6 tbsp aquafaba
- 1/8 c. melted Earth Balance
- 1/8 c. vegetable oil
- Pinch of salt
- ½ a mashed banana
- 1 tsp vanilla and agave (optional)

PREPARATION

1. Preheat the oven to 400F.
2. Mix all of your dry ingredients together.
3. Add remaining wet ingredients and mix well.
4. Mix in mashed bananas thoroughly.
5. Oil muffin pan and add in about ¾ of the way. Muffins will rise, so do NOT fill the batter all the way to the top.
6. Bake for 10 mins, then pull muffins out drizzle agave on top and then place back in.
7. Bake for another 10 minute or until golden brown.
8. Garnish with cinnamon and butter.
9. Serve after the muffins cooldown for 5 minutes.
10. Enjoy!

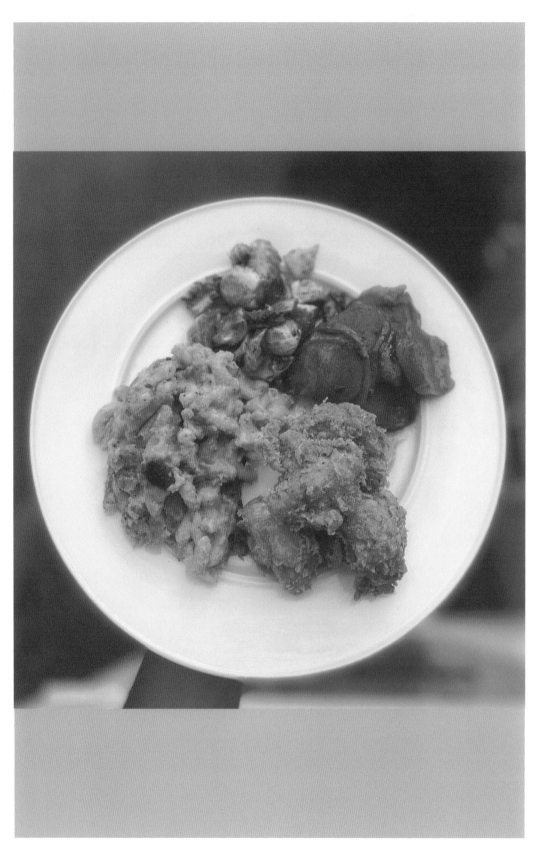

SOUTHERN FRIED CHIKIN

PREP IN
25 minutes

READY IN
20 mins

SERVES
4 person

TIPS

- Adjust seasonings to your liking.
- Best results with a deep fryer.
- Oyster mushrooms can be used for this.
- Make sure batter is not too thick or it will come out doughy.
- Longer you soak cauliflower in salt water the better the flavor.
- Substitute flour for your choice. Garbanzo bean flour is another favorite of mine.

INGREDIENTS

- 1 c. unbleached all purpose flour
- ½ - ¾ c. non dairy milk
- 1 ½ c. seasoned flour (dry mix)
- 1 tbsp garlic powder
- 1 tbsp seasoned salt
- 1 tsp onion powder
- 1 tsp cumin
- ½ tsp dried thyme
- ½ tsp cayenne
- 1 tbsp paprika
- Half a bottle of cooking oil (vegetable, peanut, etc), for frying.
- Head of cauliflower
- 1 tbsp arrowroot powder
- Healthy pinch of salt and pepper

PREPARATION

1. Prep Cauliflower into bite sized florets and cut off stems. Soak in salt water for 15-30 minutes.
2. Pour oil into a deep fryer and let it heat up. Usually takes 10 minutes.
3. Mix flour, dry seasonings, and non dairy milk, together until you reach a batter consistency. Similar to funnel cake batter. Set to the side.
4. In a separate bowl mix together dry batter with paprika and a heavy pinch of salt, arrowroot powder, and garlic powder **ONLY**.
5. While your oil is heating up, start the battering process. One hand will be your dry hand and one hand will be your wet hand. With your wet hand place cauliflower in the batter until coated thoroughly. PLACE ON A RACK OR LET IT "DRAIN" for about thirty seconds so it gets an even coating. Do that to each piece of cauliflower.
6. With your DRY hand take the cauliflower and coat with seasoned flour.
7. Drop in oil and let the cauliflower cook for 5-7 minutes or until golden brown for the best results.
8. Enjoy!

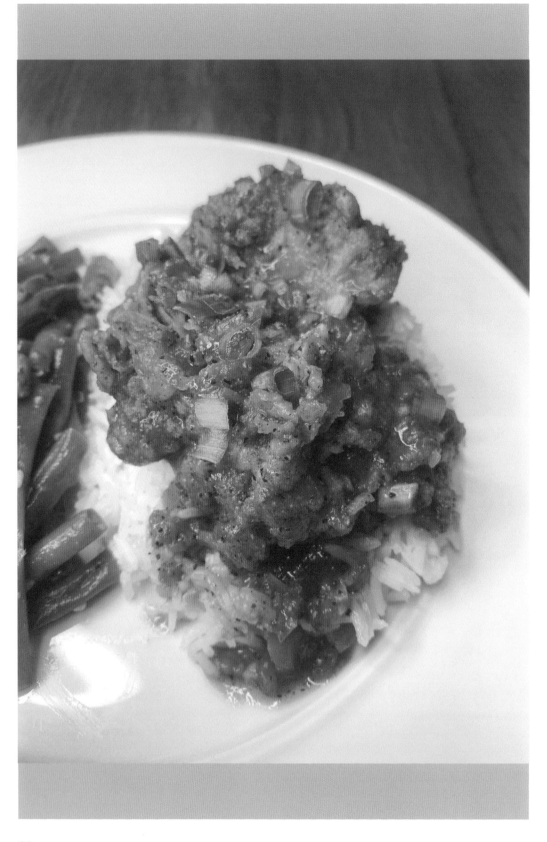

SMOTHERED CHIKIN

PREP IN
15 minutes

READY IN
30 mins

SERVES
4 People

TIPS

- Adjust seasonings to your liking.
- Best results with a deep fryer.
- Baking this will work too.
- Make sure batter is not too thick or it will come out doughy.
- Longer you soak cauliflower and mushrooms in salt water the better the flavor.
- Seasoned flour = 1 tbsp paprika, 1 tbsp cajun seasonings, ½ tsp thyme, 1 tbsp garlic powder, pinch of pepper.
- Substitute flour for your choice. Garbanzo bean flour is another favorite of mine.

INGREDIENTS

- 1 c. unbleached all purpose flour
- ½ - ¾ c. non dairy milk
- 1 ½ c. seasoned flour (*see tips*)
- 1 tbsp garlic powder
- 1 tbsp cajun seasoning
- 1 tsp onion powder
- ½ tsp cumin
- ½ tsp cayenne
- 1 tbsp paprika
- Cooking oil (vegetable, peanut, etc), for frying.
- Head of cauliflower
- 1 pack of oyster mushrooms
- Rice
- 1 tbsp arrowroot powder
- Healthy pinch of salt and pepper

PEPPER GRAVY

- 1 green onion, diced
- ¼ cup celery, diced
- ½ onion, diced
- 3 garlic cloves, minced
- 16 oz vegetable stock
- 1-2 tbsp on flour
- 1 tbsp vegan butter
- 1 tsp paprika

- 1 tsp garlic powder
- ½ tsp onion powder
- ¼ tsp red pepper flakes
- Heavy pinch of pepper
- Pinch of salt

PREPARATION

1. Prep Cauliflower and oyster mushrooms into bite sized pieces and cut off stems. Soak in salt water for 15-30 minutes.

2. Mix flour, dry seasonings, and non dairy milk, together until you reach a batter consistency. Similar to funnel cake batter. Set to the side.

3. In a separate bowl mix together dry batter with paprika and a pinch of cajun seasoning, arrowroot powder, and garlic powder **ONLY**. Set aside.

4. For the gravy add minced garlic, onion, celery, and onion to a well oiled pan on medium heat. Cook for 3-5 minutes or until translucent. If it starts to stick add a little bit of water to your pan. Season veggies with a pinch of salt and pepper.

5. Add in 1 tbsp of flour and vegan butter to create a roux. Coat all of the veggies with the flour and add in the vegetable stock along with all of the dry seasonings listed under **Pepper Gravy.**

6. Bring to a simmer and wait for the gravy to thicken up. If the gravy does not thicken up after 5-7 minutes mix flour and veggie stock in a separate bowl and then add it to the gravy to help it thicken. Leave the gravy on low and stir every few minutes.

7. Pour oil into a deep fryer and let it heat up. Usually takes 10 minutes.

8. Prepare rice based on package instructions.

9. While your oil is heating up, start the battering process. One hand will be your dry hand and one hand will be your wet hand. With your wet hand place cauliflower and oyster mushrooms in the batter until coated thoroughly. PLACE ON A RACK OR LET IT "DRAIN" for about thirty seconds so it gets an even coating. Do that to each piece.

10. With your DRY hand take the cauliflower and coat it with seasoned flour.

11. Drop the cauliflower and mushrooms in the oil and cook for 5-7 minutes or until golden brown for the best results.

12. Place the "chikin" in the pepper gravy and allow it to soak up the flavor. Do this with EACH piece.

13. Serve over rice. Garnish with gravy and green onions.

14. Enjoy!

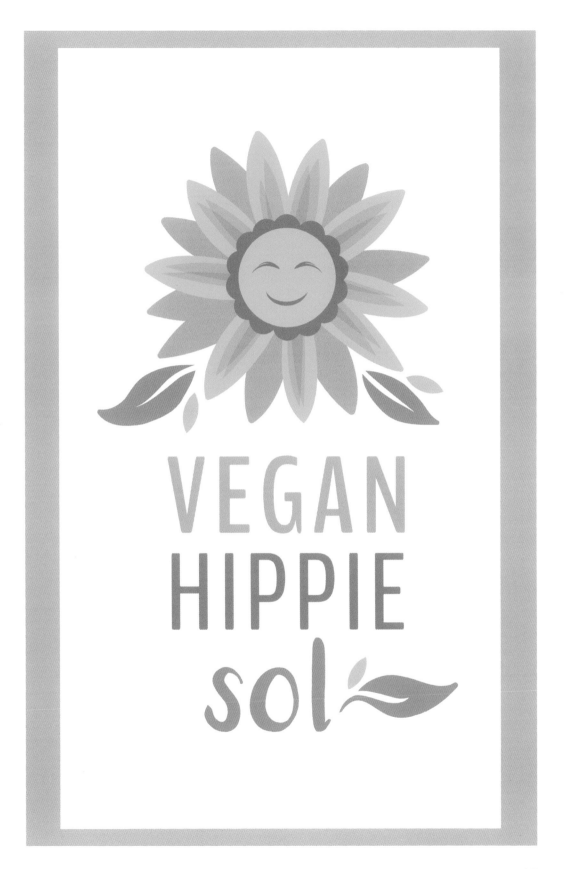

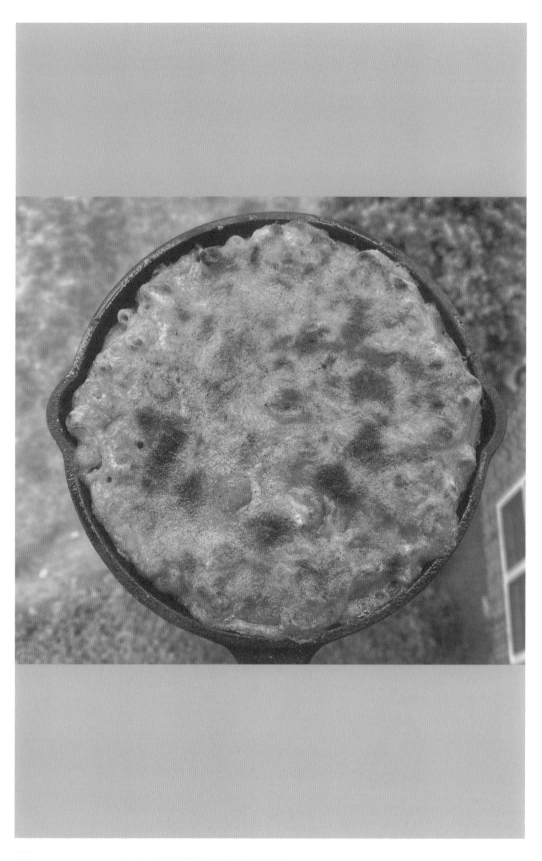

SOULFUL MAC N CHEEZ

PREP IN
45 minutes

READY IN
40 mins

SERVES
4-6 People

TIPS

- Adjust seasonings to your liking.
- The more milk you add the more seasoning you'll need to add on top because it will cook out when you bake it.
- Cornstarch can be subbed for Arrowroot powder.
- The more cheese sauce the better, so it will retain moisture and creaminess.
- Better to over-season cheese sauce than under-season. Taste cheese sauce before putting it on noodles.
- For a creamier consistency add 2 tbsp of plant-based cream cheese to your sauce and let it melt on the stove.

INGREDIENTS

- 2 tbsp nutritional yeast
- 1 tsp cayenne
- 1 tbsp garlic powder
- 1 tbsp onion powder
- 1 tsp black pepper
- 1 ½ tbsp seasoning salt
- 1 tbsp smoked paprika
- 1 tsp himalayan salt (optional)
- 1 ½ tsp mustard seed powder (optional)
- Half cap of apple cider OR lemon juice
- ½ c. cashews
- ½ -¾ c. sweet baby carrots
- 1/2 -1 c. non-dairy milk
- 1 yukon gold potato
- 3 garlic cloves or minced garlic
- 1 tbsp arrowroot powder
- ¼-½ cup daiya cheese (optional)
- 1 teaspoon of liquid smoke (optional)
- 1 box of macaroni noodles
- 3 tbsp earth balance butter

PREPARATION

1. Prepare all vegetables. Roast carrots and potatoes and garlic cloves in olive oil and salt on 400 for 20 minutes or until soft. Add ¼ cup of water half way through the roasting process.

SOULFUL MAC N CHEEZ

This will help create steam, so the vegetable can soften.

2. Boil cashews for 10 mins or until soft.

3. In a food processor add potatoes, cashews, carrots, garlic cloves, arrowroot powder, and all of the seasonings in.

4. Slowly add milk and blend it until smooth. Add lemon juice or apple cider vinegar.

5. Boil your noodles, strain, and set aside. Under cook them a tad, because it will cook more in the oven. Preheat your oven to 375 fahrenheit.

6. Season noodles with butter and salt in the same pot you boiled them in. When the butter is all melted pour in half of your cheese sauce to coat noodles and allow the arrowroot and daiya to do its job. Add in your plant-based cream cheese. (Once heated it will help create a cheesy consistency. DO NOT PUT THE BURNER ABOVE LOW/MEDIUM or it will over cook the cheese sauce).

7. Pour coated noodles into a pan or cast iron skillet to bake. Add in the other half of your cheese sauce and mix. You want to completely cover the noodles with the cheese sauce.

8. Top with paprika, butter, and parsley, vegan cheese (optional). Cover and bake on 375 for 10-15mins.

9. After baking, remove the cover and broil on high for two minutes or until the top is crispy.

10. Enjoy!

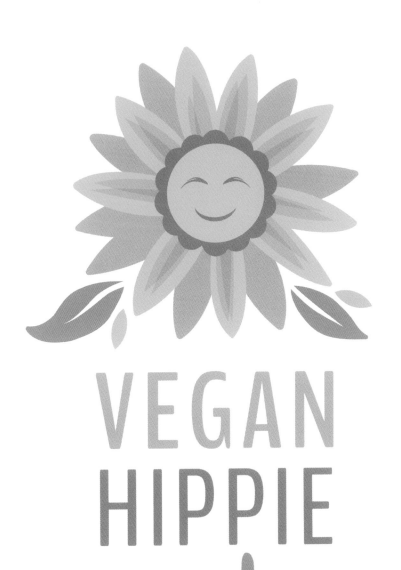

VEGAN
HIPPIE
sol

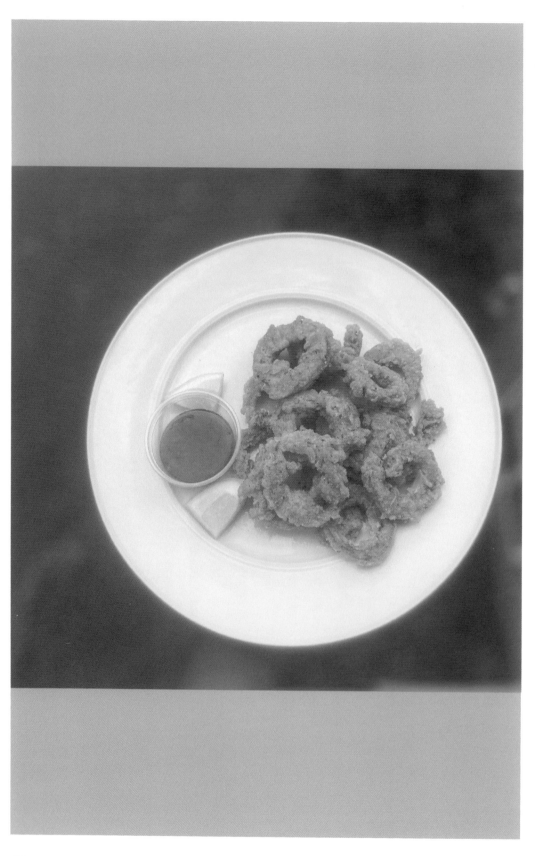

BANGIN' CALAMARI

PREP IN
20 minutes

READY IN
25 mins

SERVES
6 People

TIPS

- Make batter thinner than funnel cake batter, but thicker than a runny liquid. If you do not do this, the better will be too doughy.
- Use seasonings that you like.
- Use Peanut oil or any frying oil.
- Ripples Pea Milk (Unsweetened) is **recommended**.
- Don't over think. Cooking should be fun.

INGREDIENTS

- 4 king oyster mushrooms
- 1 tbsp old bay seasoning
- 1 tsp smoked paprika
- 1 tsp pepper
- Pinch of salt for taste
- 1 package of vegan seaweed
- Crushed parsley for garnish
- 1 lime
- 1 c. vegetable stock
- 1 tbsp soy sauce
- Frying oil

FLOUR DREDGE INGREDIENTS

- 1 ½ -2 c. flour
- 1 tbsp old bay
- 1 tbsp garlic powder
- 1 tbsp onion powder
- 1 tsp chili powder
- 1 tsp turmeric
- 1 tsp cumin
- 2 tbsp paprika
- Salt and pepper to taste
- ½ -1 c. non-dairy unsweetened milk
- 1 ½ c. of all-purpose flour

PREPARATION

1. Cut oyster mushrooms like scallops and then take a small cookie cutter and cut a hole in the middle of the mushroom. Should look similar to onion rings.

2. Mix veggie broth, soy sauce, and half a pack of seaweed in a bowl. Place mushrooms inside the marinade. Cover with a lid and set aside for

30 minutes.

3. In a separate bowl, mix together salt, pepper, and 1 tbsp paprika.

4. In a separate bowl mix together flour, dry ingredients, and your plant-based milk. Be sure to SLOWLY add in your plant-based milk. The consistency should be a little thinner than funnel cake batter.

5. Heat up frying oil.

6. Now, it's time to start the battering process. Use one hand to carefully dip the oyster mushroom ring into the wet mixture, then drop it into the flour mixture. Use your other hand (it should be dry) to coat it completely. Dip it back into the wet mixture, and again into the dry mixture, keeping one hand devoted to wet and one to dry.

7. Carefully lower the twice coated oyster mushroom into the frying oil. Repeat with the remaining mushrooms until the pot is semi-full. Fry for 3-5 minutes or until crisp.

8. Continue to cook the remaining mushrooms.

9. Garnish with parsley and crushed *vegan* seaweed. Serve hot and enjoy!

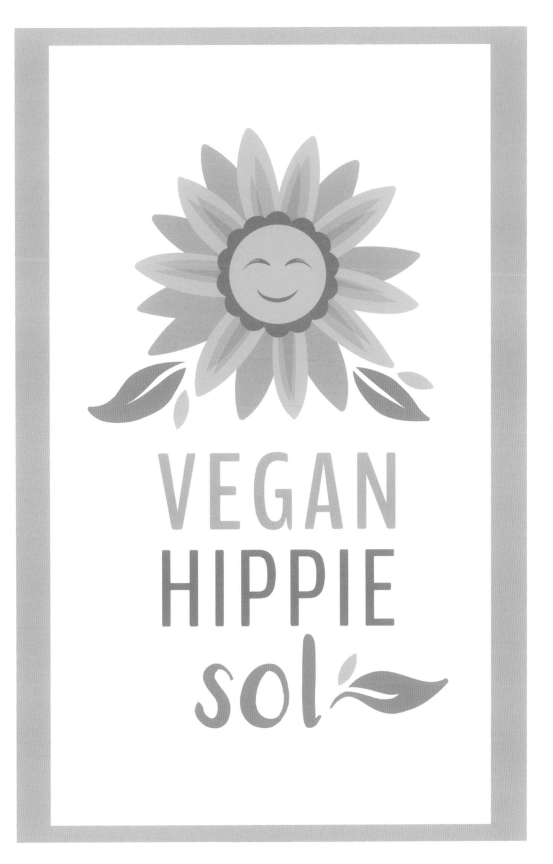

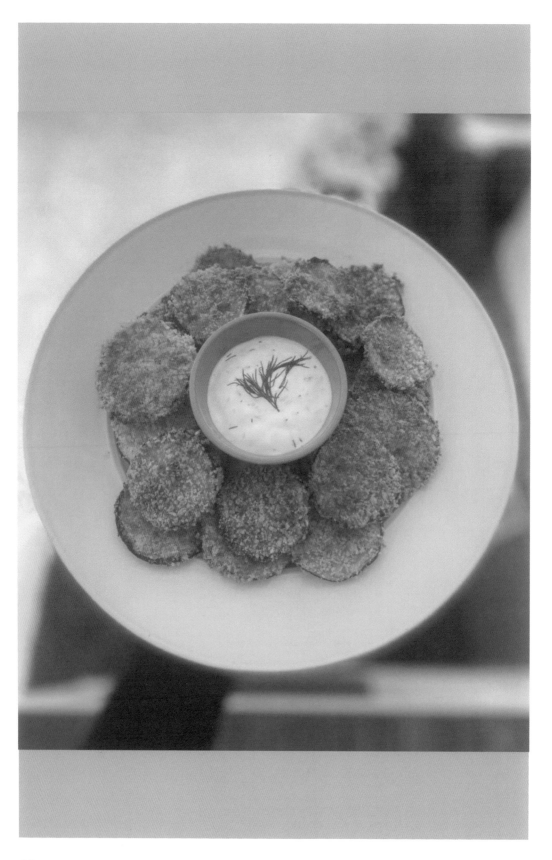

ZUCCHINI PARMESAN BITES

PREP IN
15 minutes

READY IN
20-25 mins

SERVES
4 People

TIPS

➡ Quick vegan ranch = vegan mayo, vinegar, almond milk, dill.

➡ Any egg replacer will work for this.

➡ Adjust seasonings to your liking.

➡ Feel free to add vegan parmesan to your mix.

Ingredients

➡ 1 LARGE zucchini or 2 medium zucchini

➡ ¼ cup bread crumbs

➡ ⅛ cup nutritional yeast

➡ 1 tsp garlic powder

➡ ¼ cup aqua faba or any egg replacer

➡ 1 tbsp olive oil

➡ Salt

➡ Pepper

PREPARATION

1. Preheat the oven to 425 degrees F.

2. Slice zucchini into ¼-½ inch rounds. In a bowl combine zucchini, oil, aquafaba, nutritional yeast, garlic powder, salt, and pepper. Coat evenly and set aside for 10 minutes.

3. After the zucchini sits for 10 minutes add bread crumbs in and coat evenly. If the bread crumbs aren't sticking add in more oil.

4. Bake for 20-25 minutes or until golden brown.

5. Enjoy with some vegan ranch!

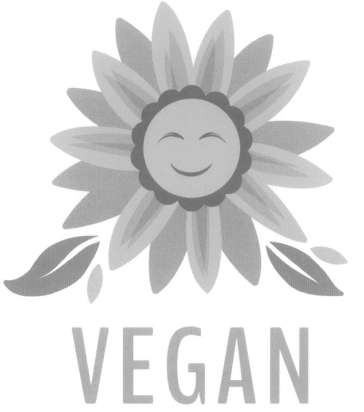

VEGAN HIPPIE

sol

PEACHIN' COBBLER

PREP IN
15 minutes

READY IN
60 mins

SERVES
6-8 People

TIPS

- Evenly spread the peaches throughout the batter.
- Canned peaches and frozen peaches work best.
- Drain the first can of peaches completely. Drain second can of peaches half way. Leave half of the syrup and use it.

INGREDIENTS

- 1 c. all-purpose flour
- 1 c. coconut sugar
- 1 c. almond milk
- 2 cans peaches
- 1 tbsp. cinnamon
- 1 tsp. Nutmeg
- 1 ½ tsp Baking powder
- Pinch of salt
- 1 tsp. Vanilla
- 1 tsp. Agave
- ½ c. Earth Balance

PREPARATION

1. Preheat the oven to 350.
2. In a large pot on medium temperature add peaches, cinnamon, nutmeg, vanilla, and agave and stir in everything evenly. Simmer for 30 minutes.
3. In a mixing bowl sift in dry ingredients and mix thoroughly.
4. Mix in almond milk and vanilla.
5. Melt Earth Balance butter and pour into an 8x8 baking pan. Make sure it covers the bottom of the pan.
6. Pour in wet batter followed by the peaches. Spread peaches evenly through the batter.
7. Bake in the oven for one hour.
8. Let the peach cobbler cool for 20-40 minutes and then serve with your favorite vegan ice cream on top.
9. Enjoy!

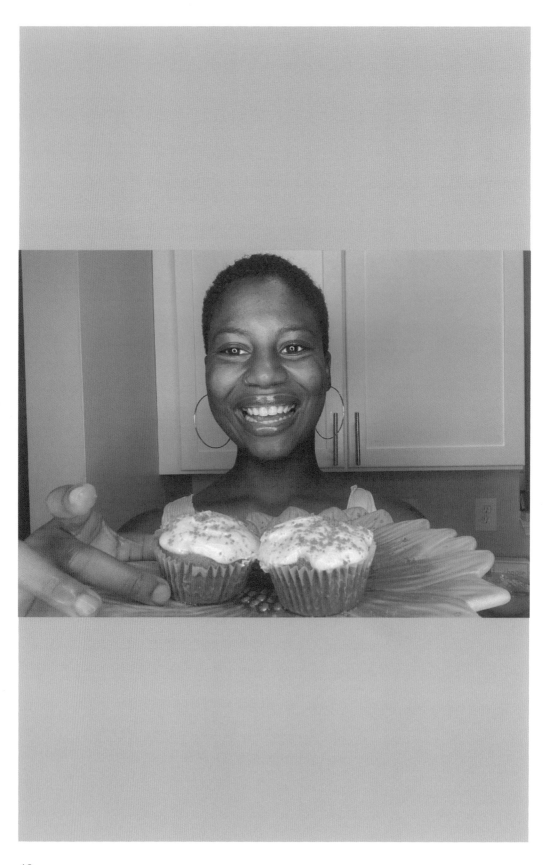

BISCOFF CUPCAKES

PREP IN
15 minutes

READY IN
60 mins

SERVES
6-8 People

TIPS

→ Most egg replacers will work for this recipe if you don't have access to aquafaba.
→ Biscoff can be found at any major grocery stores.

INGREDIENTS

→ Cupcakes:
→ 1 and 1/2 cups Unbleached All Purpose Flour
→ 1 cup Brown Sugar
→ 1 tsp Baking Soda
→ 1/2 tsp Salt
→ 1 cup Almond Milk
→ 2 tsp Maple Syrup
→ 1/4 cup Biscoff Cookie Butter
→ 1/3 cup vegetable oil
→ 6 tbsp aquafaba (chickpea juice)

FOR FROSTING

→ 2-3 cups powdered sugar
→ 1-2 tsp Almond Milk
→ 4-6 tbsp Vegan Butter
→ 1/4 cup Biscoff Butter (optional)

→ **FOR TOPPING**

→ Crumbled biscoff cookies

PREPARATION

1. Preheat the oven to 350 degrees F.

2. Sift flour into a large mixing bowl and then add in all dry ingredients. Mix together

3. Add your wet ingredients to your dry ingredients except for the biscoff butter. Mix until combined. Careful not to overmix.

4. Add in the biscoff butter and mix until combined. Taste your butter and adjust sweetness to your preference.

5. Line cupcake trays with liners and spray with cooking spray. Fill each cupcake liner up until it's about 3/4 full.

6. Bake for 20-22 minutes. Once the toothpick comes out clean they are finished. Let cupcakes cool for 30 minutes.

7. Prepare your frosting by combining all ingredients and mixing with an electric mixer until fluffy. Place frosting in the fridge or freezer while cupcakes are cooling. DO NOT LEAVE ICING OUT!

8. Decorate your cupcakes with icing and biscoff crumbs and enjoy :)

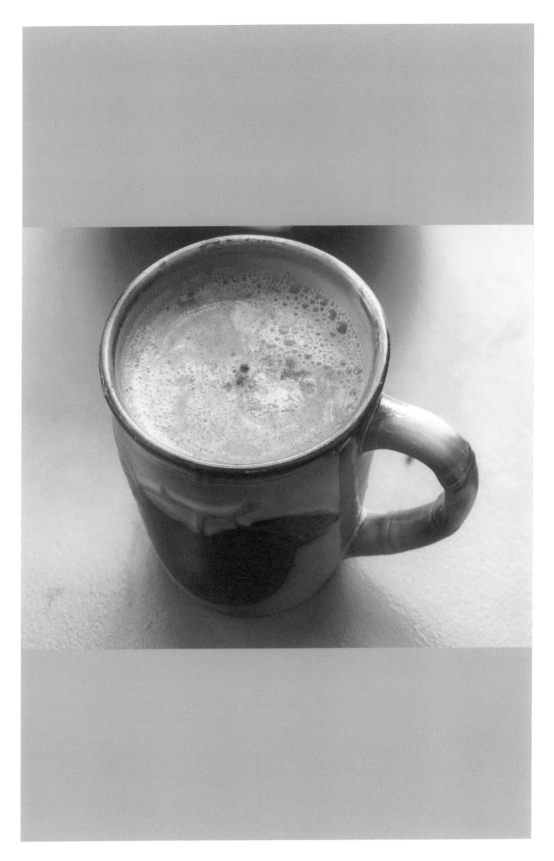

VEGAN GOLDEN MILK TEA

PREP IN
2 minutes

READY IN
8 mins

SERVES
3-4 People

TIPS

→ Do NOT skip out on the black pepper. That step is NOT optional. The black pepper activates the turmeric and allows you to receive the benefits from the turmeric.

→ Adjust agave to preferred level of sweetness.

→ Turmeric helps reduce cardiovascular complications, prevents cancer, and boosts immune functions.

INGREDIENTS

→ 3 tsp of Turmeric

→ 1 ½ tsp Black Pepper

→ 2 ½ c. unsweetened almond milk

→ 2 tsp cinnamon

→ 2 tsp agave

→ 1 tsp nutmeg (optional)

PREPARATION

1. In a small saucepan mix together turmeric, almond milk, and agave on medium low heat

2. Bring to a simmer and then add cinnamon, pepper, and nutmeg. Let simmer for another 2-3 minutes.

3. Garnish with cinnamon or coconut whipped cream.

4. Enjoy!

VEGAN HIPPIE'S GROCERY LIST:

FRUITS/VEGETABLES

- Oyster mushrooms
- Portobello mushrooms
- Chanterelle mushrooms
- White mushrooms
- Shiitake Mushrooms
- Baby carrots
- Cauliflower
- Green peppers
- Red peppers
- Sweet onions
- Yellow onions
- Yukon Gold Potatoes
- Celery
- Garlic
- Corn
- Banana's

SPICES

- Garlic powder
- Turmeric
- Thyme
- Pepper
- Cayenne
- Paprika
- Onion powder
- Salt
- Season salt

- Bay Leaves
- Cumin
- Chili pepper flakes
- Mustard powder
- Chili powder
- Old bay
- Nutritional yeast
- Coconut sugar
- Cinnamon
- Vanilla

VEGAN ALTERNATIVES

- Beyond ground beef
- Almond milk
- Daiya cheese
- Coconut milk
- Earth balance
- Vegetable stocks
- Beyond Sausage

NUTS

- Cashews

OTHER

- All purpose flour
- Agave
- Yellow corn maize
- Olive oil

VEGAN HIPPIE'S GROCERY LIST:

- Vegan BBQ sauce
- Aquafaba (chickpea juice)
- Grits
- Macaroni noodles

RECOMMENDED APPLIANCES

- Instantpot
- Deep fryer
- Ninja food processor
- Chef's knife
- Cast Iron skillet
- Standard pots and pans

ACKNOWLEDGEMENTS

To my mother, Montina: Thank you for always encouraging me to follow my dreams and laying the foundation for my soulful roots. Thank you for always cooking two meals for our family and supporting Lera's vegan lifestyle! I love you to the moon and back!

To my siblings, Lera and Mansir: I am so grateful for your never-ending support! Thank you Lera for introducing our family to the plant-based lifestyle over the past ten years. Without you none of this would be possible. There is no **Vegan Hippie Sol** without our family.

To my friends; Ulises and Dalton: Thank you for being a wonderful taste tester as I experimented night after night. I love cooking because of all of you! Cooking for you has truly been a dream come true. Y'all make me laugh and continue to inspire me daily. Without y'all these recipes could not reach the max potential. Thank you from the bottom of my heart!

To my **Vegan Hippie** supporters: I really consider you all family. Thank you for never ending support and for showing to each event and for buying this book! Writing this book has been a dream come true.

To my team: Thank you for believing in **Vegan Hippie Sol**! Thank you for the countless edits, cover changes, and overall production of the book! I appreciate your hard work.

Finally to my ancestors: Thank you for laying the foundation for soul food. Without my ancestors blood, sweat, and hard work none of this wouldn't be possible. I hope to make you all proud one day with my vegan soul food!

"As a brand Vegan Hippie wants to eliminate the stigma surrounding veganism and introduce a plant-based way of life to more people without judgement. 100% vegan - 100% affordable - 100% made with love."

Printed in Great Britain
by Amazon